Natural Beauty Secrets

The Best Natural Beauty Recipes for a Naturally Beautiful
You

By: Cassandra Green

9781681279169

Publishers Notes

Speedy Publishing LLC

40 E Main Street, Newark, Delaware, 19711

Contact Us: 1-888-248-4521

Website: http://www.speedypublishing.co

REPRINTED Paperback Edition: 9781681279169

Manufactured in the United States of America

Dedication

This book is dedicated to my friend, Abby. Who's beautiful inside and out.

Table of Contents

Chapter 1- Discovering the Truth About All Natural Beauty

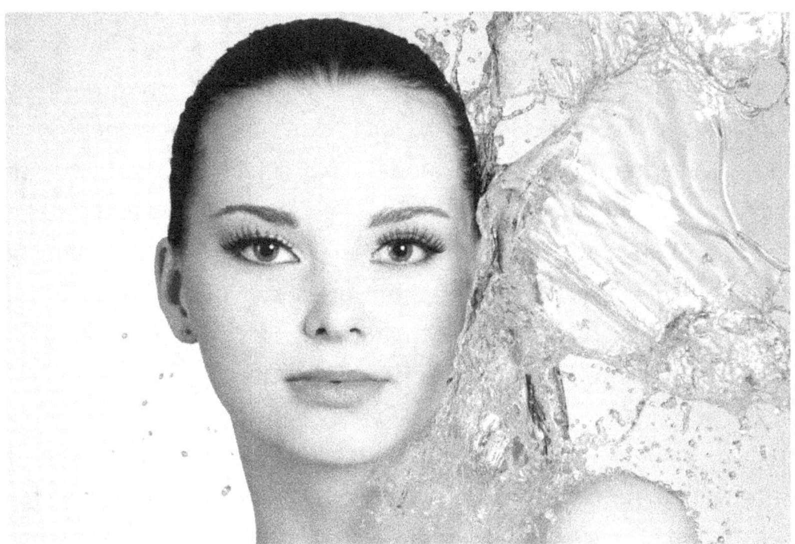

All natural beauty is something many women want but few know they have. Instead, they get expensive surgeries done, literally risking their lives in the pursuit of a beauty standard that is not only unrealistic but is completely unreal. They use beauty products that damage their skin and hair and ultimately wind up in landfills when they don't have the promised effects. Women are hurting themselves and the environment all in an effort to be beautiful.

Fortunately, there are many different ways women can achieve the all natural beauty that they so desperately want and deserve. Some of these ways are exceptionally easy to incorporate into a woman's everyday life. Some of them may be a little bit trickier for some to get used to doing everyday but once fitted into a woman's daily habits, they will be easy to maintain for a lifetime.

The first step to all natural beauty is to stop idolizing the models you see in magazines or on billboards. Nearly all advertisements in magazines, billboards, even head shots used in portfolios, have been touched up in one way or another digitally to get rid of wrinkles, acne, or other unsightly blemishes. No woman can ever live up to how a model looks in a photo because the photo simply isn't real.

Next, women everywhere need to realize how beautiful they already are. Everyone has flaws or imperfections that they don't like about themselves; even models and celebrities. You need to quit focusing on where you think you don't measure up and instead focus on things you like about yourself. For some women, finding things they appreciate about themselves can be a difficult task. Recruit friends and loved ones to tell you what they like about you. You don't have to restrict yourself to looks, either.

Which leads to the next truth about all natural beauty: it comes from within. It may sound very cliché but the phrase has existed for a long time for a reason. People with picture perfect bodies but who have ugly hearts and souls may lead a charmed life on the outside but on the inside; things aren't as lovely.

Because they are so mean and hurtful to those around them, they drive people away from them, and wind up alone in the end.

Surround yourself with people that are truly beautiful from the inside and you will not only be happier but you'll stop turning to a Hollywood standard that even models and celebrities can't live up to. Don't be tempted to turn into a plastic person through plastic surgery or other extreme measures in order to be a fantasy version of someone who doesn't know you exist. The truth about all natural beauty is in understanding the beauty within.

Chapter 2- Guide to Natural Skin Care

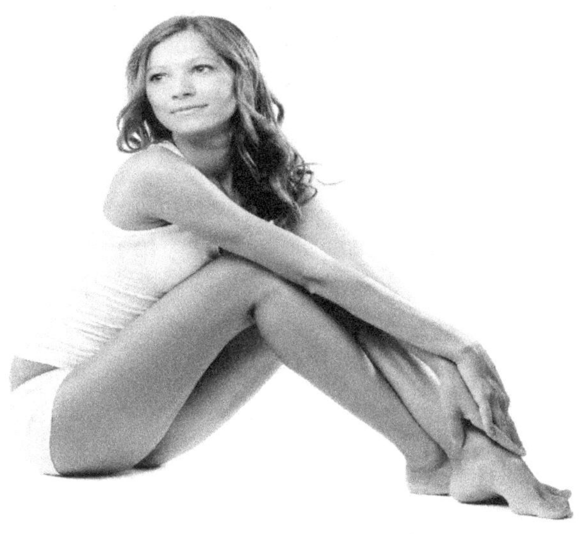

Natural skin care products may be the answer if you are concerned about the chemicals in most commercial cosmetic products. Some of these chemicals may be toxic enough to actually accelerate the aging process, which is the opposite of what you are trying to accomplish with your skin care. Even in these days of increased regulation and consumer watchdog groups; there are a number of new products introduced each year that still contain damaging chemicals.

Almost nine hundred toxic chemicals have been found in commercial cosmetic products by the National Institute of Occupational Safety and Health. The Cancer Coalition has stated that cosmetic and personal care products pose a higher threat of cancer than even smoking cigarettes. Compounding the problem is the vast amount of incorrect information distributed by marketing departments to attract new customers.

Everything that you put on the surface of your skin is absorbed into the pores and gets into the bloodstream. The circulation of the blood distributes the toxins throughout the entire body, causing damage to internal organs as well as the skin. Since all of these products enter your body, you should analyze the labels on your cosmetic products the same way you would with labels on food. Of course, choosing only natural skin care products eliminates the problem of toxins altogether.

Once the toxins get into your bloodstream, it forces your body to work much harder than usual in an effort to get rid of them. The liver is responsible for most of this clean up, but it can only handle so much before health problems will set in. The liver is a key part of the body's immune system and should be treated with care. Liver problems can cause major health issues such as auto-immune diseases, asthma, continual infections, and allergies.

Using natural ingredients can avoid these toxicity problems. The body recognizes natural skin care products as organic matter to be processed, not as a toxic threat that must be eliminated. Many of these products are made out of plant matter which contains the same basic vitamins and minerals as the ones already present in our bodies. Synthetic chemicals may be seen by the body as toxic and the immune system will react against them.

You can exfoliate with a gentle material such as crushed oatmeal, table sugar, or baking soda. Make exfoliating a regular part of your daily skin care routine and you will see much more life and bounce in your appearance. Other natural substances that may be useful for skin care include honey, egg whites, olive oil, bananas, and avocado. Be creative and use of some of the common items you have in your kitchen to give you softer, smoother skin.

How do you know which natural skin care products are actually safe? Some products are labeled as "100% natural" when they still contain chemicals and toxins. The only way to be completely sure is to look at the list of ingredients on the package. Dyes, fragrances, and synthetic preservatives can all be found in these "natural" skin care products. Women everywhere around the world are literally dying to know natural beauty secrets. As women go under the knife for one plastic surgery after another, they risk their lives and their bodies in an attempt to appear naturally beautiful. Little thought is given to how a botched surgery can affect them or their loved ones down the road. All they can think of is this unrealistic image of what's considered beautiful that they have in the heads thanks to the media and advertising.

The truth is, natural beauty secrets are not really all that secret. Everywhere a woman looks, she can find all natural ways to become someone that is truly beautiful instead of trying to imitate a digitally airbrushed and otherwise changed photograph from an ad in a magazine. A couple of the biggest secrets entail nothing more than loving yourself for precisely that you are, perceived imperfections and all.

If you're a happier person, your interactions with others will be more pleasant. If you treat others more kindly, they will also be happier. The world could literally be a better place if women decided to love themselves; instead of aspiring to be something no normal woman could ever be.

Everyone wants a better quality of life. For some women, they feel that if they just looked like that model or such-and-such celebrity, they would have everything they could possibly want and more. They feel that sort of beauty will open doors for them. In reality, while beauty might open a few doors, those doors will quickly be shut if you're ugly on the inside. A woman who is dedicated to getting what she wants and feels she deserves will go much farther in this world than one who relies on her good looks alone.

Another benefit of the natural beauty secret of being happy with who you are, at the end of the day, when all is said and done, you only have yourself. If you don't like yourself as a person, you can't expect anyone else to like you, either. While some may immediately be drawn to you because of your perceived beauty, they will quickly leave once they realize how poisonous your personality is. You'll wind up alone, with only a mirror for company.

Stop letting others dictate what you should wear, how you should look, or how you should act! Don't let people who don't even know you tell you what to do with your life and body! The media and advertising executives don't know who you are. They don't even know you exist. Make the choice to do what's best for you. That is the real natural beauty secret.

Chapter 3- Natural Beauty Tips to Help You Look Your Best

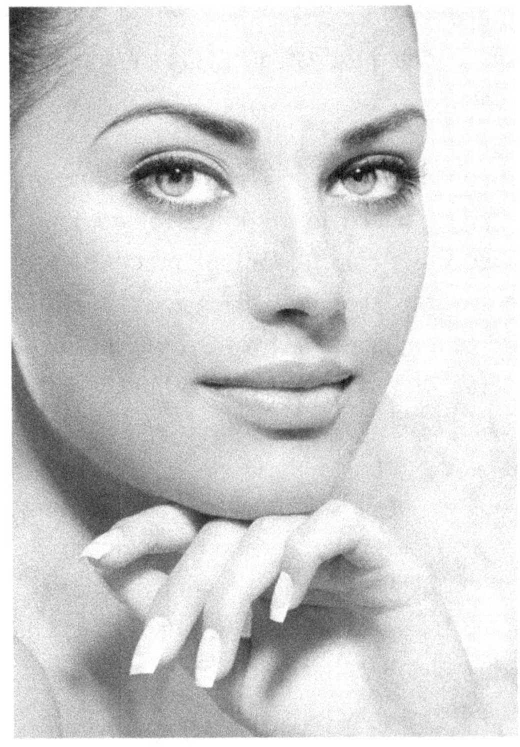

Let our natural beauty tips help you look beautiful without all those toxic chemicals found in today's cosmetics. It is possible to achieve a healthy, vibrant appearance using only natural ingredients. You'll look better and feel better because you do not have all those heavy cosmetic products on your skin.

Natural beauty refers to a vital and healthy look for your body, hair, and skin. Living an overall healthier lifestyle is the first step to refreshing your appearance. Take care of your body from the inside out before attempting to fix skin problems with surface treatments like moisturizer or makeup. Many times, a simple lifestyle change is all it takes to completely revitalize your look.

Make sure you are eating right and are getting enough vitamins and minerals each day. Add a multivitamin to your morning routine to ensure that you are receiving all the nutrients your body needs. Eat plenty of fruits and vegetables and try to avoid excess fats, sugars, and processed foods. Healthy food for your body will show through in your appearance as your skin clears and becomes more moist and supple.

Exercise is probably the most powerful of any of the natural beauty tips. Regular physical activity improves blood flow to the skin, giving it a fuller, more colorful look naturally. Of course, exercise will also help you stay trim and looking good all-around. On top of the benefits to your appearance, working out on a regular basis will keep your internal organs and heart healthy, along with preventing some cancers and extending your life.

The next in our list of natural beauty tips is to always keep you hydrated. As skin dries out, it becomes inflexible and more susceptible to wrinkles. Instead of applying heavy moisturizing cream externally, try drinking more water to provide moisture from the inside. This is a far healthier and natural solution to the common problem of dry skin.

Even if you still want to wear some cosmetics, there are natural beauty tips that can help you. Start off with either a sheer foundation or a slightly tinted moisturizing cream. Use a damp sponge to apply the cream so you get coverage all over your face without too much cosmetic buildup. This shows off your healthy-looking skin, but will also cover up any blemishes or marks without being too heavy or obvious.

To avoid leathery, dry skin, stay out of the sun whenever possible. The UV rays from the sun will dry out your skin and cause it to wrinkle prematurely. If you must go out in direct sunlight, be sure to wear sunscreen that is rated SPF 15 or higher. Hats, sunglasses, and umbrellas can also help protect you when you are out in the sun.

As you can see it does not require chemical-filled cosmetics and makeup to look great. There are many ways to enhance your appearance without resorting to artificial products. Following these natural beauty tips will get you on your way to a healthier, more radiant appearance.

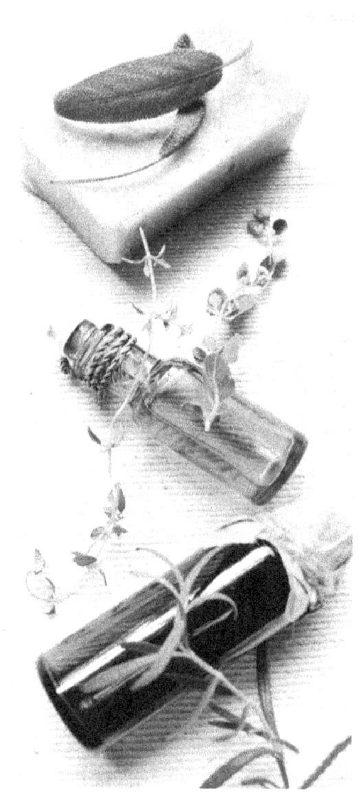

Apple Tart Soap
Ingredients:
4oz. Clear, Unscented Glycerin Soap
1 Tablespoon Liquid Soap
1 teaspoon Liquid Glycerin
1/2 teaspoon Apple Fragrance Oil
2 Drops Red Food Color
1/2 teaspoon Ground Cinnamon
Melt soap in small pan over low heat or in a glass cup in the microwave. Add Liquid Soap and glycerin and stir gently but well. Add fragrance, color and cinnamon. Stir and let stand a couple minutes, just enough to start to thicken so when you stir again the cinnamon will be more evenly distributed. Pour into molds. Allow

setting completely (in or out of freezer). Wrap in plastic wrap or use cellophane candy bags.

Apricot Freesia Tarts
Ingredients for Tart:
1 lb White Glycerin Soap Base
12 Drops Cosmic Color Canary Yellow
11 Drops Cosmic Color Red
1 t. Apricot Freesia FO
Ingredients for "Whipped Cream" Topping:
4 oz White Glycerin Soap Base
¼ t. Apricot Freesia FO
A "Shake" of Super Sparkle Gold Sparkle Dust TM
Melt soap base for tart in a double boiler. Once melted, add color and fragrance. Pour into a muffin tin and allow hardening. Remove from tin. Melt soap base for topping and add a shake of Sparkle Dust. Using with an electric mixer, mix until thick and bubbly. Spray tarts with rubbing alcohol and spoon the topping onto the tarts while allowing some to run over tarts. Top with a dash of Sparkle Dust if desired.

Aspen Dreams Bath Salts
Ingredients are:
2 cups of Epsom salts (or a mixture Epsom/sea)
2 tablespoons of baking soda
Essential oils:
5 drops of rosewood
2 drops cedar wood
2 drops Chamomile
A nice jar with a tight fitting lid
To make the salts:
Mix the salts and baking soda in a bowl very well.
Mix oils in a small cup. Take them and pour them evenly over the salt. Mix the two very well. Let it sit for over an hour before placing in a jar and sealing. For coloring these use yellow and red to make a light brown.

Balancing Bath Salts

Ingredients:
Sea Salt--3 tbsp
Baking Soda--3 tbsp
Essential Oils--8 drops
Jar--4 oz

Choose 3 or 4 oils from these essential oils: Bergamot, Frankincense, Geranium, Lavender, Palmarosa, Rose, and Rosewood. Add sea salt, baking soda and oils to jar. Gently shake to mix, mix well. Add to tub of running water.

Balancing Red Earth Salts

Ingredients:
Sea Salt--2 tbsp
Baking Soda--3 tbsp
Powdered Red Earth Clay--1 tbsp
Essential Oils--8 drops
Jar--4 oz
Choose 3 or 4 oils from these essential oils: Bergamot, Frankincense, Geranium, Lavender, Palmarosa, Rose, and Rosewood. Add sea salt, baking soda, powdered red earth clay and oils to jar. Gently shake to mix, mix well. Add to tub of running water.

Balancing Seaweed Salts

Ingredients:
Sea Salt--2 tbsp
Baking Soda--3 tbsp
Powdered Kelp--1 tbsp
Essential Oils--8 drops
Jar--4 oz
Choose 3 or 4 oils from these essential oils: Bergamot, Frankincense, Geranium, Lavender, Palmarosa, Rose, and Rosewood. Add sea salt, baking soda, powdered kelp and oils to jar. Gently shake to mix, mix well. Add to tub of running water.

Basic Bubble Bath

Ingredients:

5 drops fragrant oil or essential oil (your choice)

1 quart water

1 bar castile soap (grated or flaked)

1 1/2 ounces glycerin

Directions:

Mix all ingredients together. Store it in a clean container. Pour in running water.

Basil and Lime Bath Salts

Ingredients:

You will need:

5 cups of Sea Salt (or Epsom salt, or a combination of both)

1 Tsp. of Baking Powder

2 Tsp. of Almond Oil

5 drops Lime Scented Oil

4 drops Basil Oil

1 drop green coloring

1 drop yellow coloring

All you have to do is mix the salt and the baking powder in a bowl. In a smaller bowl mix together all liquids and add to salts, stirring well. You should let them sit so they can soak up the scent and the coloring all of the way through. After they have sat for about two hours take them and place them in jars with cork stoppers. To create a good seal dip the cork in melted wax (green to match salts) and put cork into bottle.

Bath Cookies

Ingredients:

2 cups finely ground sea salt

1/2 cup baking soda

1/2 cup cornstarch

2 tbs. light oil

1 tsp. vitamin E oil

2 eggs

5-6 drops essential oil

Preheat oven to 350 F. Mix together all the ingredients. Take a teaspoon of the dough and roll it gently into a ball about 1" in diameter. Continue doing this with all the dough and place the balls on an ungreased cookie sheet. (You can decorate the cookies with clove buds, anise seeds, or dried citrus peel if you wish.) Bake the cookies for 10 minutes, until they are lightly browned. Do not over bake. Allow the cookies to cool completely. To use, drop 1 or 2 cookies into a warm bath and allow dissolving. Do not eat! Yield: 24 cookies, enough for 12+ baths.

Bath Bombs
Ingredients:
2 tbs. citric acid (you can get this at a pharmacy)
2 tbs. cornstarch
1/4 cup baking soda
3 tbs. coconut oil (or any other emollient oil like almond, avocado or apricot kernel oil)
1/4 tsp. fragrance oil
3-6 drops of food coloring (if desired)
Paper candy cups
Place all of the dry ingredients (first 3) into a bowl and mix well. Place coconut oil into a small glass bowl and add fragrance and food coloring. Slowly add oil mixture into dry ingredients and mix well. Scoop up small amounts of the mixture and shape into 1" balls. Let the balls rest on a sheet of waxed paper for about 2 to 3 hours, then place each ball into a candy cup to let dry and harden for 24 to 48 hours. Store bombs in a closed, air-tight container. To use, drop 1 to 3 bombs into warm bath water.

Bubble Bags
Ingredients:
Used in the shower, when there is no time to take a soaking bath.
2 parts oatmeal
2 parts dried herbs
1 part grated soap
Place ingredients in a cloth bag and use as a washcloth
15. Candy Cane Bath Salts
Ingredients:
3 cups of Epsom salts
3 Teaspoons of Sweet Almond Oil
9 drops of Peppermint Essential Oil

1 drop of red food coloring (more if you like)
1 drop of green food coloring
To decorate: several jars with turn lids or cork seals red, green and white Christmas ribbon several gift tags shaped like candy canes OR Several candy canes (small ones) to make the salts separate each of the three cups of salts into three bowls. Separate each teaspoon of almond oil into three bowls. Into one bowl of almond oil add the drop of red food coloring; into the second add the green. Into each of the three bowls of oil add three drops of peppermint oil. Mix each bowl well. After mixing pour each of the bowls of oils and coloring into one of the bowls of salt. This will leave you with a bowl of green a bowl of red and a bowl of white scented salts. Let sit for a few hours covered. To create the candy cane effect layer layers of each color, a layer of red, a layer of green , a layer of white, over and over until you fill the jar.

Chamomile Fields Shampoo
Ingredients:
4 bags of chamomile tea (or 1 handful of fresh chamomile flowers)
4 tbs. pure soap flakes
1-1/2 tbs. glycerin
Let the tea bags steep in 1-1/2 cups boiled water for 10 minutes. Remove the tea bags and with the remaining liquid add the soap flakes. Let stand until the soap softens. Stir in glycerin until mixture is well blended. Pour into a bottle. Keep in a dark, cool place.

Champagne Bubble Bath
Ingredients:
1/4 C foaming concentrate
3/4 C distilled water
1/2 tsp. table salt (not sea salt)
1 TBSP. glycerin
1/4 tsp. Champagne or white wine fragrance oil
Buy a split of champagne- drink it or toss it but keep the bottle. Heat water (not boiling just hot), stir in concentrate and glycerin until completely dissolved. Add fragrance oil and stir well. Add salt stirring until dissolved. Allow mixture to cool. If it is not as thick as you would like add another 1/4 tsp. salt stirring until dissolved. Pour into a clean champagne split and seal bottle. Using a pink or

white paint pen create labels for the front and back on gold stickers. With a square of candy foil cover the cork, twisting at the neck.

Chocolate Soap

Ingredients:

12 oz grated soap

5 oz water

1/4 cup instant cocoa powder

1/8 oz Chocolate Fragrance oil

Combine the grated soap and water in a saucepan, and set on medium heat. When the soap has melted, add the cocoa powder, and chocolate fragrance. Stir well, and then pack into molds and let sit until hardened.

Citronella Soap

Ingredients:

1 cup grated Castile soap

1/2 cup water

10 drops citronella essential oil

5 drops eucalyptus essential oil

1 T. dried, crushed pennyroyal leaves

Mix the ingredients into the melted soap/water mixture. With an electric mixer, whip the soap until it has doubled in volume. Spoon the soap into the prepared molds, pushing it into the molds as best you can (the beating action cools the mix, so work quickly). If the mixture has cooled off and thickened so much you can't put it into the molds, hand mold the soap into large balls.

City Shampoo (Removes Impurities from Hair)

Ingredients:

3/4 cup distilled water

1/4 cup shampoo concentrate (or substitute with 1/2 cup unscented shampoo and increase salt to 1 tsp.)

1/2 tsp. table salt

1 tbs. dried thyme

1 tbs. dried peppermint

1 tbs. dried lavender

1 tsp. witch hazel

1 tsp. almond oil

7 drops cinnamon oil

3 drops ylang-ylang oil

Cassandra Green

This shampoo is known to be effective in removing impurities such as smog and city grime from the hair. In a heavy saucepan, bring the water to a boil and add the dried thyme, peppermint and lavender. Remove the pan from the heat and let steep for 30 minutes. Strain the herbs from the water and pour the herbal infused water into a ceramic bowl. Add the shampoo concentrate and stir until well mixed. Add the salt, witch hazel, almond oil, cinnamon oil and ylang-ylang oil to the mixture, stirring until thick. Bottle and close.

Cold Cream Soap

Ingredients:
4 oz M&P soap
2 tsp cold cream
10 drops fragrance oil
1 drop coloring (optional)
Melt soap, then add cold cream and stir until melted. Remove from heat; add fragrance and color, and then mold.

Cranberry Bubble Bath

Ingredients:
8 oz. unscented liquid soap
2 oz. distilled water
7 drops bergamot oil
5 drops lime oil
3 drops vanilla fragrance oil
2 drops gardenia fragrance oil
Mix all together and pour into a container.

Chocolate Cookie Soap

Ingredients:
1 lb. Opaque MP
1 Tbsp. Cocoa butter
Cocoa powder for colorant (or brown dye)
1 Tbsp. Chocolate FO
Round or cookie molds
Melt the MP soap. Remove from heat and slowly stir in the cocoa butter and enough cocoa powder to make it a pale brown or tan. Add fragrance oil. Reserve enough of the soap to make a darker

brown color. Pour the lighter shade of brown soap into round/cookie molds. Add more cocoa powder to the reserved batch of MP base to make a darker brown.

Cinnamon Soap

Ingredients:

4 oz. MP base

10 drops cinnamon oil

1 drop red food coloring (optional)

Melt MP base. Remove from heat and stir in the cinnamon oil and coloring until well mixed. Pour the soap into a mold and let set for three hours.

Coffee & Cream Soap

Ingredients:

1 4oz. bar Glycerin soap

1 teaspoon ground espresso

1 teaspoon powdered milk

10 drops coffee fragrance oil

In a small saucepan over low heat, melt the bar of glycerin soap until liquefied. Remove from heat and stir in ground espresso, powdered milk, and coffee fragrance oil. Pour soap into a mold and let set for three hours or until hardened.

Coffee and Cream Soap 2

Ingredients:

2 tsp. Coffee beans (can replace with 1 tsp. instant espresso)

4 oz. MP base

1 tsp. Heavy whipping cream

1 tsp. Aloe Vera gel

Grind two teaspoons of your favorite coffee beans to espresso grade in coffee grinder. Melt the MP. Remove from heat and add the ground coffee, whipping cream, and Aloe Vera gel, and stirring until well blended. Pour the mixture into a mold and let set for three hours or until hardened.

Creamsicle Soap

Ingredients:

8 oz. MP base (divided into 4 oz. quantities)

10 drops orange oil

1 drop orange food coloring

3 Tbsp. Heavy whipping cream

10 drops vanilla fragrance oil

Melt soap and remove from heat. Add the orange oil and food coloring, stirring until well mixed. Pour half of the mixture into each soap mold and let it set for an hour. When the orange soap has set, melt the second half of MP base. Remove from heat and stir in the whipping cream and the vanilla fragrance oil. Pour the melted soap into the molds on top of the orange soap. Let it set for three hours. Your finished bars should come out half orange and half white.

Cucumber Loofah Soap

Ingredients:

3 oz. opaque soap

2 tsp. powdered loofah

15 drops cucumber fragrance oil

1 T. Aloe Vera gel

Green coloring

Mold

Shred the soap in a food processor and set aside. Boil 1/2 cup of water over low heat and stir in the shredded soap. Continue stirring until the mixture becomes a sticky mass, approximately four minutes. Remove from heat and stir in the Aloe Vera gel, the fragrance oil and the coloring until well blended. Spoon the mixture into a mold and let set for six hours or until hardened. Wrap finished soaps in cellophane.

Custom - Scented Bath Crystals

Ingredients:

Rock salt or sea salt (you can also use water softener salt for this; it is much cheaper than sea salt)

Essential oils

½ quart glass or clear plastic jar with tight-fitting lid

Add approximately 4 teaspoons of the essential oil to the rock salt in a ½ quart container. If container is larger or smaller, add or subtract oil as needed. Cap the lid tightly and wait at least two days before using.

Custom - Scented Bath Oil

Ingredients:

Sunflower oil

Essential oil or potpourri refresher oil in your choice of scent(s)
Corked container
Crystal beads, dried flowers, little seashells, etc. (optional - for bottle decoration)
Pour sunflower oil through a funnel into the corked container, leaving a little space at the top, at least an inch. Add 4 teaspoons of the essential oil per 1/2 quart. Cork the container and agitate the bottle gently. Let it sit for 2 to 3 days before using. You may add things to the container to make it as pleasing to the eye as it is to the nose... whatever you want or will match the decor of your bathroom.

Custom - Scented Bath Powder

Ingredients:
1/2 cup cornstarch
2 tbs. arrowroot powder
2 tbs. baking soda
Few drops of essential oil of your preference
Combine ingredients in a bowl and mix well. Let stand a few days to dry, and then sift through a flour sifter. Pour into a powder shaker / container.

Custom - Scented Shampoo

Ingredients:
3/4 cup distilled water
1/4 cup shampoo concentrate (or substitute with 1/2 cup unscented shampoo and increase salt to 1 tsp.)
1/2 tsp. table salt
20 drops fragrance oil of your choice
Food coloring of your choice (optional)
Warm the water and pour into a ceramic bowl. Add the shampoo concentrate and stir with a wire whisk until well blended. Add the salt, fragrance oil and food coloring and stir until well blended. Pour into a bottle and close.

Custom - Scented Shower Gel

Ingredients:
1/2 cup unscented shampoo
1/4 cup water

3/4 tsp. salt
15 drops fragrance oil
Food coloring (optional)
Pour shampoo into a bowl and add the water. Stir until it's well mixed. Add the salt, fragrance oil and food coloring. Suggestions for scents: kiwi extract, raspberry extract, strawberry extract, coconut extract, vanilla extract, etc... (I personally like the raspberry and vanilla mix.

Deep Conditioner for Beautiful Hair
Ingredients:
1 small jar of real mayonnaise
1/2 of an avocado
Put ingredients together in a medium bowl and squish together with your hands until it's a minty green color. Smooth into hair all the way to the tips. Put on a shower cap or wrap your head with saran wrap. Leave on for 20 minutes. For deeper conditioning put a hot, damp towel around your head over the shower cap or saran wrap. If you have really long hair and only need conditioning at the ends, cut the ingredients in half and apply only to the ends and just wrap them.

Desert Sands Layered Bath Salts
Ingredients:
5 drops yellow food coloring
4 drops red food coloring
4 drops musk oil
3 drops Jasmine fragrant or essential oil
3 cups Epsom salts
1 cup baking soda
2 tsp. glycerin
Combine baking soda, Epsom salt and glycerin until well blended. Add scents until there are no clumps, just a fine powder. Divide the mixture evenly into 3 separate bowls. In the first bowl add 3 drops yellow food coloring, in the second bowl add 3 drops red food coloring, and in the third bowl add 2 drops yellow food coloring and 1 drop red food coloring. Stir each bowl until the color is well mixed. Allow the air to dry it for a few hours before placing in a

bottle. Once dried, layer the colors... red first, then orange, then lastly yellow.

Detox Bath
Ingredients:
Place in warm tub of water:
Epsom salts--2 handfuls
Organic sea salt--1 handful
Sweet Almond Oil--2 teaspoons
Rosemary--4 drops
Violet Leaf--4 drops

Dry Shampoo
Ingredients:
1/2 cup cornstarch
Fragrance oil (optional)
Sprinkle cornstarch into your hair and massage into hair and scalp. Allow it to absorb for a few minutes, and then brush through hair. Repeat if necessary. This is wonderful to freshen-up your hair in a pinch between shampoos... or great to take on camping trips when fresh water is unavailable for using a liquid shampoo. You can also add a couple drops of fragrance oil to the cornstarch for a nice scented dry shampoo.

Earth Angel Bath Crystals
Ingredients:
1/2 cup Epsom salts
3/4 cup baking soda
1/2 cup sea salt
2 tsp. almond oil
20 drop patchouli oil
15 drops cypress oil
5 drops rose oil
Green food coloring (one or two drops)
Mix it all together very well. Sometimes it helps to add wet together separately in another bowl before adding to baking soda and salts. You will need to use a few heaping tablespoons to your tub to use

Chapter 5- Homemade Natural Lotion for Your Skin Type

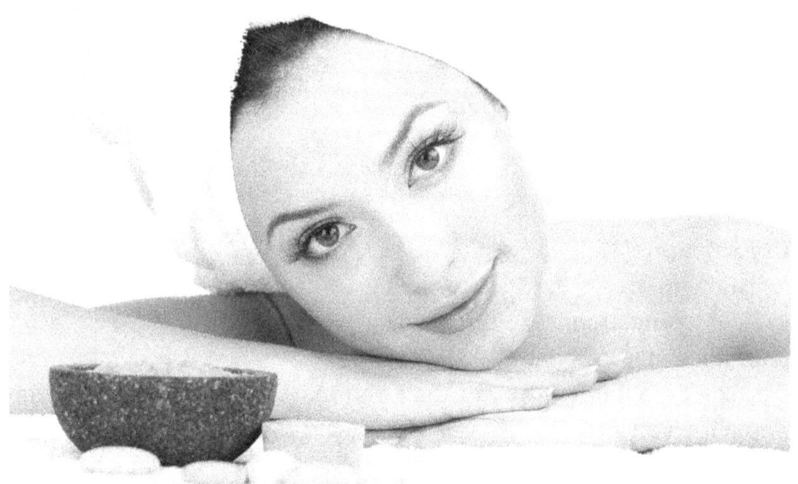

Almond Orange Body Lotion
Ingredients:
1/8 tsp. borax powder
1/2 c. almond oil
1 tsp. coconut oil
1 tsp. grated beeswax
2 tbsp honey.
3-4 drops essential orange oil
Make as for Mint Body Lotion

Almond Oil Wrinkle Cream
Ingredients:
1 tbs. of an infusion of comfrey leaves or
1 tbs. of a decoction of comfrey roots
1 tbs. lanolin
2 tsp. sweet almond oil
2 tsp. water
2 tsp. cod liver oil
Melt lanolin and almond oil in a double boiler. Add water and allow cooling. Mix in cod liver oil and comfrey. Apply gently to face and rinse off after 5 to 10 minutes. This is a rich moisturizer that boosts

the water-holding capacity of your skin and helps plump out wrinkled areas. Infusion: This is a beverage made like tea, by pouring boiled water over plants and steeping to extract the active ingredients. The normal amounts are about 1/2 to 1 ounce of plant to one pint of boiled water. You should let the mixture steep for 5 to 10 minutes, covered, and strain the infusion into a cup. Decoction: This preparation allows you to extract primarily the mineral salts and bitter principles rather than vitamins and volatile ingredients. The normal amounts are about 1/2 ounce plant to 1 cup water. Bring ingredients to a boil, then reduce heat and simmer for up to 4 minutes. Remove from heat and steep the mixture with the cover on the pot for a few minutes.

Almond Rosewater Body Lotion
Ingredients:
1/4 cup rosewater
1/4 cup glycerin
2 tbs. witch hazel
1 tbs. almond oil
Mix together rosewater and glycerin. Add witch hazel and almond oil. Stir completely to dissolve. Pour into a pretty bottle. Recipe for rosewater: To prepare rosewater, first gather fresh rose blossoms; do this during the morning, after the dew has evaporated. Place the petals in a glass, stainless steel, or enamel saucepan and cover them with distilled water. Weigh the floating petals down with a heat-resistant glass dish. Place the pan over low heat and allow the pot to release steam for at least an hour. You should begin to see drops of rose oil floating on the surface of the water. Do not allow the water to boil. When the water has taken on a rosy hue, feels thick and soft, and shows evidence of rose oil on its surface, strain the liquid through a tea strainer, using your fingers to press all the liquid from the petals. Store it in refrigerator. Rosewater may be used as a skin toner; just apply to the face with a cotton ball. Important Notes: NEVER use rose petals that have been sprayed with any kind of pesticide for making rosewater!! Consider using only enough distilled water to cover the rose petals. Otherwise, the solution becomes more dilute. Please remember to use only the petals, not the sepals, stamens, or green foliated bracket holding the petals in their grouping.

Apricot Butter Cleansing Cream (For Dry Skin)

Ingredients:

10 oz apricot kernel oil

2 oz cocoa butter

2 oz beeswax

Heat all in top of double boiler until wax and butter are melted. Beat with a wooden spoon until smooth and cooled. Transfer to jars, cap and refrigerate.

Apple- pear nighttime wrinkle lotion

Ingredients:

1 tsp apple juice

1 tsp lemon juice

1 tsp lime juice

2 Tbsp buttermilk

1TBSP rosemary leaves

3 seedless grapes

1/4 pear

2 egg whites

Blend all ingredients on medium speed for 30 seconds using a cotton ball, dab mixture on areas around the eyes and wherever wrinkles have developed. Let dry, then rinse with warm water. Use no more than 3 times a week. Follow with a moisturizer. Cover and refrigerate immediately, discard after 4 days.

Avocado Eye Cream

Ingredients:

5 drops almond oil

3 ripe avocado slices

Blend almond oil into avocado. Dab around eyes and leave on for 5 minutes, and rinse.

Beach Sand Foot Scrub

Ingredients:

2 Tablespoons Canola oil

2 Tablespoons beach sand

3-5 drops rosemary oil

Combine and mix into a paste using a fork. Massage scrub onto feet, concentrating especially on problem areas. Rinse off with warm water and pat dry.

Beeswax Hand Cream
Ingredients:
¼ cup beeswax
¼ cup almond oil
¼ cup honey
1 tablespoon bee pollen
¼ cup Vaseline petroleum jelly
¼ cup glycerin
2 tablespoons liquid lecithin
Melt the beeswax and petroleum jelly together over a double boiler. Add the remaining ingredients and heat for 4 to 5 minutes until the mixture is smooth and heated. Pour into a container while still hot since it will harden as it cools.

Beeswax Coconut Hand Cream
Ingredients:
¼ cup beeswax
3 tablespoons baby oil
¼ cup coconut oil
1/3 cup glycerin
Melt the beeswax and coconut oil over a double boiler. Add the remaining ingredients and heat until mixture is smooth, for about 4 to 5 minutes. Pour into a container while still hot since it will harden as it cools.

Bee Pollen Hand Cream
Ingredients:
1/2 cup petroleum Jelly
1/2 Cup glycerin
1/3 cup beeswax
2 tablespoons bee pollen
Melt the petroleum jelly and beeswax over a double boiler. Add the glycerin and heat for several minutes until the mixture is smooth and well heated. Add the bee pollen and pour into a container while still hot since the mixture does harden as it cools.

Materials needed, other than hive products, are readily available at drug stores and health stores.

Beeswax Cold Cream

Ingredients:

1/3 cup beeswax

¼ cup glycerin

1 tablespoon liquid lecithin

¼ cup baby oil

¼ cup almond oil

1 tablespoon bee pollen

Melt the beeswax over a double boiler. Add the remaining ingredients and heat for several minutes until well mixed. Pour into containers while still hot since it will harden as it cools.

Beeswax-Almond Hand Cream

Ingredients:

¼ cup beeswax

½ cup almond oil

½ cup coconut oil

¼ cup rosewater

Melt the beeswax and coconut oil over a double boiler. Add the remaining ingredients and heat until well mixed, several minutes. Pour into a container while still hot since it does harden as it cools.

Body Lotion

Ingredients:

2 cups

1 cup Aloe Vera gel

1 teaspoon lanolin

1 teaspoon pure Vitamin E oil

1/3 cup coconut oil

1/2 to 3/4 ounce beeswax

3/4 cup almond oil up to 1and 1/2 teaspoons essential oil or more to prolong scent

Place Aloe Vera gel, lanolin, & vitamin E oil in blender or food processor. Place coconut oil & beeswax in 2-cup Pyrex measuring cup, microwave on high 30 seconds, and stir with chopstick. Repeat heating in 10-second blocks until fully melted. Stir in almond oil, reheating if necessary. Run blender or processor at low to medium speed, and then pour in melted oils in thin stream as if making mayonnaise. As oil is blended in, cream will turn white and blender's motor will start to grind. As soon as melted oils are added and you've achieved mayonnaise-like consistency, stop motor, add essential oil(s) and pulse-blend. Do not over blend. Transfer cream to glass jars while still warm, as it thickens quickly.

Carolina Cleansing Cream
Ingredients:
3 T. olive oil
1/2 C. lard
Several drops peppermint extract
1/2 tsp. tincture of Benzoic
Mix well in a clean glass bottle. Apply to face with fingers. Remove with tissues. Keep in a cool place. 4 T. lemon juice Combine ingredients in a clean glass bottle. Shake well and refrigerate.

Cocoa Butter Hand Cream
Ingredients:
4 tbs. beeswax
4 tbs. cocoa butter
4 tbs. almond oil
Melt together beeswax and cocoa butter. Add almond oil. Mix completely until smooth. Pour into a pretty pot or jar. Let harden and it is ready to use or to be given as a gift.

Cocoa/Shea Butter Lotion Bars
Ingredients:
1 part beeswax
1 part cocoa butter
1 part Shea butter
1 part oil (coconut, emu, etc.)
Melt all and pour into a container or mold.

Coconut Cleansing Cream
Ingredients:
3 T. coconut oil
1 T. olive oil

1 T. glycerin
2 tsp. water
Melt ingredients together over very low heat until liquid. Remove from heat. Beat as the mixture cools to emulsify. Store in an airtight jar and keep in the refrigerator since coconut oil has a very low melting point. After use, follow with an astringent.

Coconut Oil Lotion Bar

Ingredients:
1 part beeswax
1 part coconut oil
1 part grape seed oil, apricot oil or sweet almond
1 tsp. EO per lb. of total product
1/4 part Shea/mango/cocoa butter (optional)
Melt all together and pour into a container or mold

No Cocoa Butter Lotion Bar

Ingredients:
2 parts coconut oil
1 part Shea butte
2 parts beeswax
1 1/2 parts Grape seed Oil
OR
1 part Apricot Kernel Oil
Melt all, add fragrance/essential oils if desired and pour into mold or container.

Cold Cream (For Cleansing and Soothing the Skin)

Ingredients:
52 oz. white beeswax
Ingredients:
1/2 cup almond oil
1/2 tsp. borax
1/4 cup rosewater
This recipe gives you a basic all -purpose cold cream / moisturizer, which you can add scented oils to, if you'd like. Place the beeswax in a double boiler and add the almond oil. Melt the wax over low heat, stirring constantly to combine the ingredients. Take off the heat and dissolve the borax in the rosewater and slowly pour it into

the melted wax and oil, whisking constantly. It will turn milky and thicken, continue whisking while it cools. When it reaches thick pouring consistency, pour into glass jars or china pots.

Lavender Lotion
Ingredients:
1 oz. glycerin
2 tsp. oil of lavender
Put ingredients in a clean glass bottle and shake well. Refrigerate.
213. Lemon cleansing Cream
1Tbsp beeswax
3Tbsp vegetable oil
1Tbsp witch hazel
1Tbsp lemon juice
1/8 tsp borax
6 drops lemon EO
Over low heat, gently melt beeswax in the vegetable oil. Beat for 5 minutes until mixture has a creamy, smooth consistency. In a separate pot gently warm witch hazel (I infuse lavender in the witch hazel, good for the skin) and lemon juice; stir in borax until dissolved and add to cream. Beat steadily. After the cream has cooled stir in the lemon EO. Then spoon into jars. This is good for eliminating excess oil and smoothing wrinkles. Plus the lemon gives it antiseptic qualities.

Lemon Hand Lotion
Ingredients:
1 tsp. lemon juice
2 tsp. glycerin
Use 1 teaspoon of lemon juice for every 2 teaspoons of glycerin.

Magic Lotion
Ingredients:
In small pan over water melt
3 Tbsp. safflower oil
1 Tbsp. lanolin
1 Tbsp cocoa butter
1/3 cup light mineral oil
1tsp. almond extract

Cassandra Green
In a pint jar place
2 Tbsp. water
1 Tbsp glycerin
1/4 cup plus 2 Tbsp. 70% ethanol alcohol
1 drop food or other color
When the oils are cool add to the pint jar and shake. Divide into (2) 6 oz jars. In about half an hour the lotion will separate into 3 different layers. Shake and it becomes an emulsion, let stand and it separates again. This is really pretty and feels so good.

Mayonnaise Face Cream
Ingredients:
2 fresh egg yolks
1 C. vegetable oil (sesame,
Safflower or sunflower)
1 T. wheat germ oil
1 T. herb vinegar
2 drops perfume or rose geranium oil
Beat egg yolks in cold bowl. Add oil very slowly at first. Beat with rotary beater, mixer or blender. Gradually add more oil. As mixture thickens, add vinegar and fragrance. Beat until thick. Apply to face with upward and outward strokes all over face and throat. Leave on for 20 minutes. Remove with damp cloth. Follow with skin freshener.

Milk & Honey Lotion
Ingredients:
(Instant conditioner and refresher)
1/4 C. milk or cream
1/4 C. honey
Mix milk (or cream) and honey in a small glass or enamel pan. Warm until the honey melts, then remove from heat. When it is cool enough to tolerate, apply to face and neck (or your entire body if you have time). Let it stand for 15 minutes, then rinse or shower off with warm water. The mix can be made in larger quantities, and it will keep for a week if refrigerated.

Olive Oil Cream
Ingredients:

1/2 tsp. borax
2 tsp. boiling water
4 T. petroleum jelly
4 T. olive oil
Dissolve borax in boiling water. Melt petroleum jelly and olive oil over low heat until liquid. Add borax mixture. Stir to mix thoroughly. Remove from heat. Beat as the mixture cools to emulsify.

Olive Oil Shaving Cream

Ingredients:
1/4 C stearic acid
2 Tbsp olive oil
1 C hot water
1 tsp borax
2 Tbsp grated soap
Melt stearic acid and oil in double boiler until a clear liquid form. Mix hot water, borax, and soap and stir until the borax and soap are dissolved. Pour the soap solution into a blender and blend well for about 1 minute. Slowly pour the melted stearic acid mixture into the soap solution. Blend on high until a smooth cream forms. Pour into a clean container and allow cooling completely. To use, soften your beard (or legs) with warm water and then apply the shaving cream. Use a sharp, clean razor.

Orange Lotion

Ingredients:
2 T. cocoa butter, melted
4 T. olive oil, warmed
4 T. orange juice
2 drops essential oil*
* Orange flower, if possible.
Whirl all ingredients in blender until light and fluffy. Store in a
Tightly-capped bottle or jar. This does not need to be refrigerated, but if the mixture separates, beat again.

Peaches & Cream Moisturizing Lotion

Peel and mash one very ripe peach. Strain through a sieve to extract all the juice. Mix peach juice with an equal quantity of fresh cream. Keep refrigerated.

Rejuvenating Cream

Ingredients:

1 oz. beeswax or lanolin

3 oz. almond oil

4 (400 IU) vitamin E capsules

2 drops rose oil

Combine and heat over low heat until beeswax is melted. Remove from heat and whip with a whisk until cool.

Rich Skin Cream

Ingredients:

2 1/2 oz (weight) beeswax

2/3 cup baby oil

1 tsp borax

4 oz (weight) anhydrous lanolin

3/4 cup water

Fragrant essential oil (optional)

Chemically pure borax, which is required for cosmetics, is sold by drug stores. In a microwave or double boiler melt the oil, lanolin and beeswax to 160 degrees F. Heat the borax and water in a separate container to 160 degrees F. Be sure the borax is dissolved and the wax is melted. Add the water mixture to the oil mixture while stirring briskly. When white cream forms, stir slowly until the mixture cools to 100 degrees F. Pour it into small wide-mouth jars.

Solid Massage Bars

Ingredients:

1/2 cup melted cocoa butter

10 capsules Vitamin E oil

1 T. melted coconut oil

10 drops rose oil

8 drops peppermint oil

5 drops ylang-ylang oil

Mix all ingredients. Let cool a bit, then pour into molds and let harden.

There is no need to condition the molds before pouring.

Stretch Mark Cream
Ingredients:
1/4 C cocoa butter
1 Tablespoon wheat germ oil
1 teaspoon light sesame seed oil
1 teaspoon apricot kernel oil
1 teaspoon vitamin E oil
2 teaspoons grated beeswax
1 teaspoon vanilla extract (optional)
Mix together all ingredients except the vanilla extract. Heat the mixture gently until the cocoa butter and beeswax have melted; stir well. Remove from the heat and stir in the vanilla extract, if desired. Allow to cool completely. Store it in a clean jar with a tight-fitting lid. Massage into your skin.

Suntan Lotion
Ingredients:
2 oz. salt-free mayonnaise
2 oz. black tea (brewed very dark)
Juice of 1 lemon
5 (400 IU each) vitamin E capsules
Mix mayonnaise, tea and lemon juice in a blender. Pour into a storage container and squeeze contents of vitamin E capsules into it. Keep refrigerated no longer than 1 week.

Chapter 6- Homemade Facial Masks that Give Your Skin A Radiant Glow

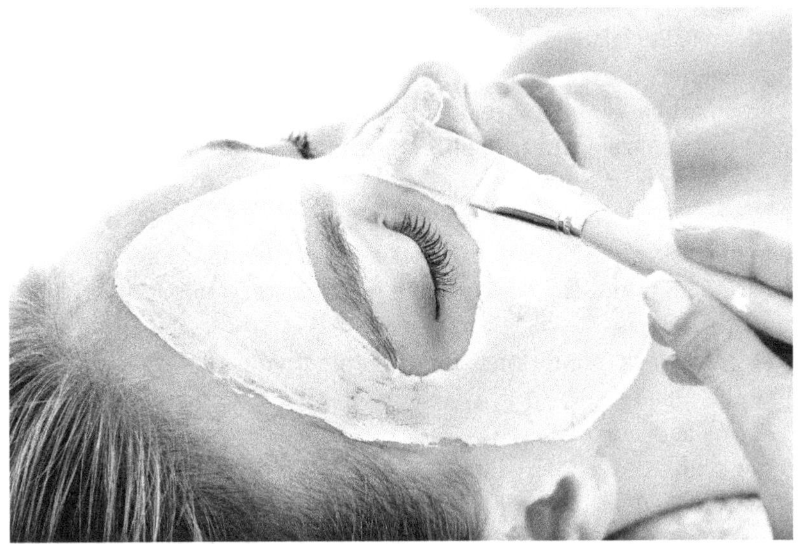

Apple Mask
Ingredients:
1 Apple, cored, quartered
2 TBSP. Honey
1/2 tsp. sage
Drop the apple slices into a food processor and chop. Add honey and sage and refrigerate for 10 minutes. Pat the mixture onto your face with a light tapping motion until the honey feels tacky. Leave it on for 30 minutes rinse off with cool water.

Apple & Honey Mask
A mask of grated apple mixed with a little honey is an excellent Remedy for pimples.

Apple Zinger Facial Mask (For Oily or Acne Prone Skin)
Ingredients:
1 medium size apple, grated fine
5 tbs. honey
Mix the grated apple and honey well. Smooth over skin and let sit for 10 minutes. Rinse off with cool water.

Apricot Mask
Mash the fresh fruit for a good face mask. Variation: Add apricots to a little warm olive oil to form a spreadable paste. Good for dry skin.

Artichoke Facial:
Ingredients:
1 fresh artichoke heart well cooked or canned hearts in water, not oil 2 tsp. light oil (avocado, olive, or canola)
1 tsp. vinegar or fresh lemon juice
In a ceramic bowl mash artichoke hearts and mix with oil and vinegar. Stir well until smooth paste. Massage on face and neck. Let sit 10 to 15 minutes. Rinse off with warm water and pat dry.

Avocado Mask (conditions and prevents dryness)
Ingredients:
1/2 ripe avocado
1 egg white
Mash avocado into a thick paste. Add egg white. Apply to face; leave on 15 to 20 minutes. Rinse with lukewarm water.

Avocado Masque (for dry skin)
Ingredients:
1/2 ripe avocado
1 tsp. vegetable oil
Mash avocado into a paste and add vegetable oil. Apply to clean skin. Leave on for 10 to 20 minutes. Rinse with warm water.

Avocado-Banana Masque (for dry or sensitive skin)
Ingredients:
1/4 mashed ripe avocado
1/2 mashed ripe banana
2 T. plain yogurt (not low-fat)
1 tsp. wheat germ oil
Mix all ingredients. Apply mixture to face and leave on 10 to 15 minutes. Rinse with tepid water.

Avocado & Honey Moisturizer Mask (For Dry Skin)
Mash up 2 tablespoons avocado, mix with 2 tablespoons honey and 1 egg yolk. Apply to face, leaving on about 15-20 minutes. Rinse with warm water. Finish with a rinse of the vinegar pH balancer.

Banana Mask
Mash a banana and spread on face for a soothing, cleansing and moisturizing face mask. Rinse clean with warm water finished with a rinse of the vinegar pH balancer.

Banana Facial
Take one banana, one cup of oatmeal, and just enough milk to create a paste. Apply to face and leave on for 10 to 15 minutes. This is great for dry skin and is also a good defoliator.

Banana Supreme Facial
Ingredients:
2 medium bananas
Honey (optional)
Mash bananas with a fork do not over mash or it will be runny. Add honey, if desired. Smooth over skin, let sit 10 minutes rinse off with cool water.

Blemished Skin Mask
Ingredients:
1 tomato, ripe, chopped
1 tsp. lemon juice
1 TBSP. instant style oatmeal or old fashioned rolled oats
Blend everything until just combined. Apply to the skin, making sure the mixture is thick enough to stay on the blemished areas. If necessary add a little more oatmeal to thicken the mask, and then scrub it off with a washcloth dipped in warm water.

Brewer's Yeast Mask (For Oily Skin)
Make a paste using the yeast and a small amount of warm water.

California Avocado Cleanser and Mask
Ingredients:
1/4 ripe avocado

1/2 C. buttermilk
1 beaten egg yolk
Blend avocado with egg yolk and buttermilk. Apply to face and throat and leave on for 5 minutes. Spread on a little more. Leave on for another 5 minutes. Rinse with tepid water.

Carrot Mask (For Oily Skin)
Carrots make an excellent skin mask for acne and blemishes.
Apply raw, grated carrots to the face while lying down, a little lemon juice may also be added.
For Cooked Carrot Mask: Boil three large carrots and mash them, or process in a food processor. Add 5 tablespoons of honey or yogurt (optional). Apply gently, in an upward motion. Leave on for 15-20 minutes. Rinse with warm water. Finish with a final rinse of witch hazel or the vinegar pH balancer.

Carrot Top Mask
Ingredients:
2-3 large carrots
4 1/2 TBSP. honey
Cook carrots, then mash with honey. Apply gently to the skin wait 10 minutes, rinse off with cool water.

Cool as a Cucumber Yogurt Facial (For Normal/Oily Skin)
Ingredients:
1/2 cucumber
1 Tbsp plain yogurt
Puree cucumber in blender. Mix in yogurt, and apply to face. Leave on for 30 minutes. Rinse well.

Corn and Oat Face Scrub
Ingredients:
1/2 cup oat flour
1/2 cup corn flour
1/3 cup whole milk powder
1/2 cup corn meal
- grind milk powder in a mortar and pestle to get the lumps out.
- sift the dry ingredients together Mix with water to get a thick paste and smooth on, splash off with water. To make the mixture

astringent use Witch-hazel To make it soothing add Aloe Gel To make it less drying for ageing or very dry skin add a few drops of Almond Oil and mix before adding final water. Note(s): Use extra fine corn meal for face scrubs and coarser grinds for body scrubs. Do not premixed with wet ingredients as this mixture will not keep if wet. I use this mixture but exclude the meal for a daily face wash.

CORNMEAL SKIN FACIAL (for oily or combination skin)
Ingredients:
1 T. dry cornmeal
2 eggs
Cleanse face, steam, splash with cool water and pat dry. Massage with the dry cornmeal. Rinse off. Then apply a mask made by whipping the eggs and brushing on face. Leave on for 20 minutes; rinse off.

Cornmeal Thigh Scrub
Ingredients:
1 small avocado stone
4 tablespoons cornmeal
2 teaspoons aloe gel
1 tablespoon cold-pressed grape seed oil
6 drops juniper essential oil
6 drops lemon essential oil
1. Put the avocado pit in a heavy paper bad, then wrap the bag around the pit a few times. With a hammer or wooden mallet, give the pit a few good whacks to break it up into smaller pieces that will fit into a coffee grinder or small food processor.
2. Grind the pieces to a gritty meal consistency. Mix the cornmeal, then place in a sterilized shallow jar, seal, and label.
3. Pour the aloe, grape seed, juniper, and lemon oils into a bowl, then sprinkle about 2 teaspoons of the avocado and cornmeal over the wet ingredients and stir. Add additional meal if necessary so that you have a gritty paste.
4. Mist your legs thoroughly with body mist, then apply the paste, using small, circular, massaging motions. Relax for 15 minutes and rinse with warm water.

Cucumber Mask {for oily skin)

Natural Beauty Secrets
Ingredients:
1/2 cucumber
1 egg white
1 T. lemon juice
1 tsp. mint
Purée ingredients in a blender and refrigerate for 10 minutes. Apply the mixture to your face and leave on for 15 minutes. Rinse with hot, then cool water.

Cucumber Mask
Ingredients:
1 cucumber, cubed
3 oz. milk
Blend together. Apply to face, and leave on for 5 minutes.

Culture Scrub
1 tablespoon table salt
1 tablespoon flavored yogurt
3 tablespoons baby oil
Mix in small bowl. Ingredient amounts can vary depending on your taste. This scrub is wonderful for winter dry skin especially where the legs are shaved repeatedly. This is not only a dead skin remover but a conditioner as well. It works well on other body parts as well. Enjoy.

Creamy Avocado Mask
Mash 1 tablespoon ripe avocado, add 1/2 tsp honey and mix. Stir in a little almond meal until creamy. Apply to clean skin, leave on for 15-20 minutes and wash off with lukewarm water. Finish with a rinse of the vinegar pH balancer.

Cucumber Mask
Ingredients:
1/2 cucumber
1 egg white
1 TBSP. lemon juice
1 tsp. mint

Puree everything and refrigerate for 10 minutes. Apply the mixture to your face and leave it on 15 minutes. Rinse with hot then cool water.

Cure-All Moisturizer

Straight olive oil serves multiple purposes. If you can't stand the smell, add a few drops of essential oil. Use as a moisturizer for dry, roughs pots on your knees and elbows. To soften cuticles, dip a cotton ball in some olive oil, dab on tops of fingernails and rub in. For a great split ends treatment, shampoo hair, use olive oil in place of conditioner on ends only, and then rinse thoroughly with warm water.

Dry Skin Face Pack

Ingredients:
4 tsp. mayonnaise
1/2 tsp. kelp powder
1 tsp. fuller's earth
Make into a paste. Apply. Leave on for 10 minutes.

Dry Skin Facial

Ingredients:
1 T. dry oatmeal
1/2 mashed ripe banana
2 oz. plain yogurt
Cleanse face, steam, splash with cool water and pat dry. Massage with the dry oatmeal. Rinse off. Then apply a mask made by mixing yogurt and banana; spread evenly on face. Leave on for 20 minutes; rinse off.

Elder Flower Mask (For Oily Skin)

Mix elder flower herb with yogurt to make a paste, apply to face.

Egg Yolk Mask

This mask is wonderful for the skin Take one beaten egg yolk and apply liberally to the face with a cotton ball. Let dry on the skin for 15 minutes then rinse off with cool water. This mask will replenish your skin and tighten up your pores.

Egyptian Facial

Ingredients:

1 egg beaten

1/2 tsp. olive oil

1 TBSP. flour

1/4 tsp. sea salt

1TBSP whole milk

Mix all the ingredients together until creamy and blended. Spread mixture face and neck. Leave on 15 minutes. Rinse off with cool water and pat dry

Enchanted Garden Mask

Ingredients:

The enzymes in the papaya help soften skin by removing dead surface cells.

1/2 papaya

1/2 tsp. lemon or lime juice

1 tsp. honey

Mash the ingredients together. Apply to clean face, leave on for 10 minutes, and rinse well.

Fruity Face Mask

Ingredients:

Bananas

Pineapples

Strawberries

Mash fruits with a fork, pat onto face and leave on 10 to 15 minutes. Rinse with cool water.

Chapter 7-Enhancing Dental Health Using Natural Care

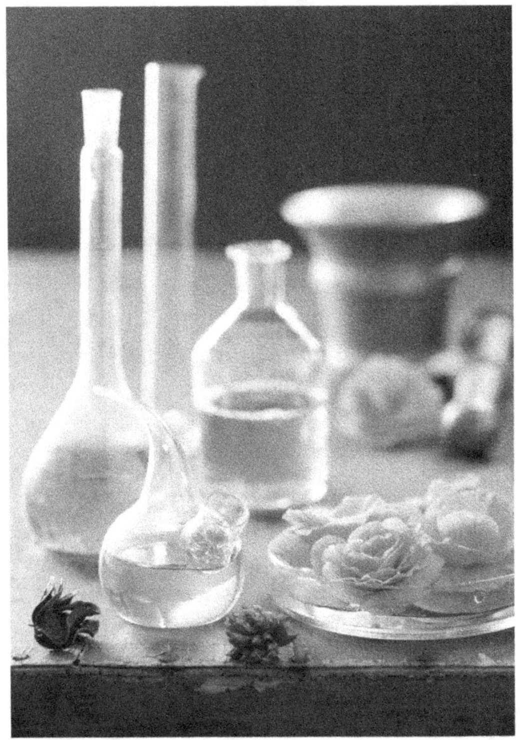

All Natural Toothpaste
Ingredients:
1/4 tsp peppermint oil
1/4 tsp spearmint
1/4 cup arrowroot
1/4 cup powdered orrisroot
1/4 cup water
1 tsp ground sage
Instructions:
Mix all of the dry ingredients in a bowl. Add water until the paste is desired the consistency. You can also substitute 1/2 tsp each of oil of cinnamon and oil of cloves for peppermint/spearmint if desired.

Breathe Fresheners
1) Chew fresh parsley to sweeten the breath.
2) Chew fennel seeds to freshen the breath.

3) Chew anise seeds to freshen the breath.

4) Chew a few peppermint or spearmint leaves or drink a cup of peppermint tea

5) Add 1 drop of myrrh oil to 1 cup of cooled, boiled water. Use as gargle/mouthwash.

Old Fashioned Tooth Powder

Ingredients:

2 Tbsp dried lemon or orange rind

1/4 cup baking soda

2 Tsp salt

Place rinds in food processor, grind until peel becomes a fine powder. Add baking soda and salt then process a few seconds more until you have a fine powder. Store in an airtight tin or jar. Dip moistened toothbrush into mixture, brush as usual.

Basic Toothpaste

Ingredients:

1 Tsp of the Old Fashioned Tooth Powder

1/4 Tsp Hydrogen peroxide

Mix into a paste and brush as usual.

Loretta's Toothpaste

Ingredients:

1 Tsp baking soda,

1/4 Tsp hydrogen peroxide

1 drop oil of peppermint

Mix to make a paste, dip toothbrush into mixture, brush as usual.

Strawberry Tooth Cleanser

Ingredients:

1 Tsp of the above Old Fashioned Tooth Powder

1 Tbsp crushed ripe strawberries

Mix strawberries and powder into a paste and brush as usual.

Vanilla & Rose Geranium Toothpaste

Ingredients:

1/2 ounce powdered chalk

3 ounces powdered orris root

4 teaspoons of tincture of vanilla
15 drops oil of rose geranium
Honey, enough to make a paste
Combine all ingredients and mix until you have a paste the consistency you like. Use a clean stick (Popsicle) to scoop paste onto brush. Store the stick in same container.

Tooth Care

1) Mash some fresh strawberries and use as you would any other "tooth paste"
2) Using fresh sage leaves, rub over the teeth to clean and whiten.

Rosemary-Mint Mouthwash

Ingredients:
2 1/2 cups distilled or mineral water
1 tsp fresh mint leaves
1tsp rosemary leaves
1 tsp anise seeds
Boil water. Add herbs and seeds, infuse for 20 minutes. Cool, strain and use as a gargle/mouthwash. If you wish to make up a larger quantity, double or triple the recipe then add 1 tsp of tincture of myrrh as a natural preservative.

Spearmint Mouthwash

Ingredients:
6 ounces water
2 ounces vodka
4 teaspoons liquid glycerin
1 teaspoon Aloe Vera gel
10-15 drops Spearmint essential oil
Boil water and vodka; add glycerin and Aloe Vera gel. Remove from the heat, let cool slightly. Add spearmint oil, shake well. Pour into bottle, cap tightly.

Chapter 8- Homemade Lip Balm and Lip Gloss for Beautiful Lips

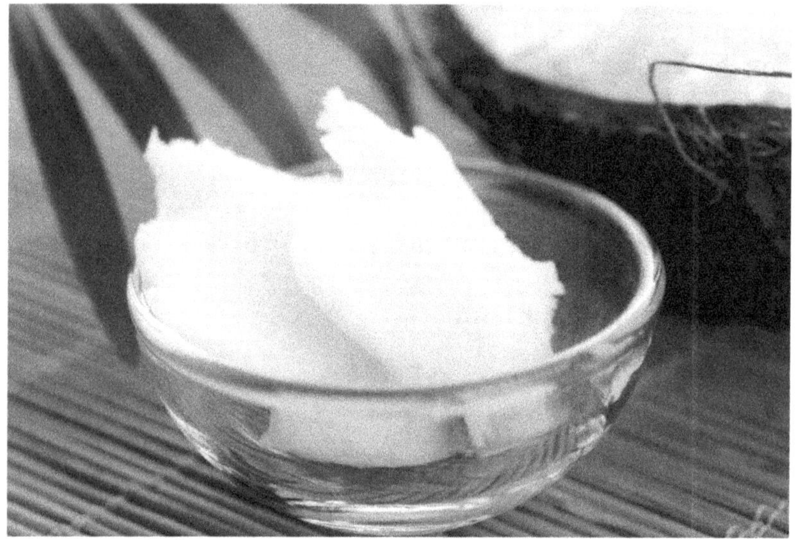

Basic Formula for Lip Balm

Ingredients:

1/4 cup vegetable or nut oil

1/4 ounce beeswax

1 teaspoon honey or glycerin (humectants)

1/2 to 1 teaspoon natural flavoring oil aka Essential Oil.

Heat the oil and beeswax in a double boiler (or microwave) until the beeswax is melted. Remove from heat and whip with an electric beater until creamy. Add the honey or glycerin and approx 5 drops flavoring oil; whip some more. Add more flavoring if desired. Store in small glass jars, small Tupperware bowls, decorative tins or film containers. Try different oils on your lips to choose the best one for your skin and taste preference. If the Balm is too hard (waxy), add more oil to your mixture. If it is too soft, add more wax. You can add a few drops of beet juice for a beautiful & natural red color. But instead of going to that trouble, you can just shave off a little of your lip stick for that beautiful (not natural) color. Don't use food coloring, it may contain alcohol base. Never use extracts found in cooking sections of the grocery stores as they contain alcohol. Use safe essential oils. The good part about them is they have thousands of great flavors. Comfrey, Rosemary, Tea Tree or Camphor Oils are excellent for healing effects. How do you know if it's time to throw away your gloss? If it changes color, odor, or texture, throw it away.

Basic Lip Gloss
Ingredients:
Paraffin wax
Coconut oil
Petroleum jelly
Candy melts (to color the gloss and make it taste sweet)
Oil-based candy flavoring (if you want a special flavor)
Grater
Wax paper
Ziploc bag
Small container

Grate a bit of paraffin wax onto wax paper. Put ¼ teaspoon grated wax into the plastic bag. Add 1 teaspoon coconut oil, 1 teaspoon petroleum jelly, and 1 candy melt to color the gloss and make it sweet. Add 1/8 teaspoon oil-based candy flavoring if you like. Seal the bag and put it in a bowl of hot water to melt the ingredients, for approximately 3-5 minutes. (Use tap water! Please never use a microwave or stove to heat the water). When all the ingredients are melted, take the bag out of the water. Move the ingredients around in bag to mix. Make sure you work quickly. Clip off a tiny corner of the bag and squeeze gloss into the clean container. Let it set for an hour. If you can't wait that long, just put this in the refrigerator for 15 minutes. Use a cotton swab to apply gloss to help your product last longer. Your lip-gloss should last a long time. If it changes color, odor, or texture, though, throw it away.

Basic Lip Balm II
Ingredients:
1/2 ounce beeswax beads, refined
4 ounces sweet almond oil
2 teaspoons essential oil or food flavoring oil
Put the 4 ounces of sweet almond oil in measuring cup, add beeswax beads and melt in microwave. Stir with spoon, and when cooled a bit, add essential or flavoring oil.
Pour into jars or containers.

Cassandra Green
Cranberry Lip Gloss
1 tablespoon sweet almond oil
10 fresh cranberries
1 teaspoon honey
1 drop of vitamin E oil
Mix all the ingredients together in a microwave-safe bowl. Microwave for a couple of minutes or until the mixture just begins to boil. (Bowl may also be heated in a pan of water on a stovetop). Stir well and gently crush the berries. Cool mixture for five minutes and then strain through a fine sieve to remove all the fruit pieces. Stir again and set aside to cool completely. When cool, transfer into a small portable plastic container or tin.

Silky Smooth Lip Balm
Ingredients:
2 Teaspoons Olive Oil
1/2 Teaspoon Grated Beeswax or Beeswax Pellets
1/2 Teaspoon Shea Butter or Cocoa Butter
1/2 Teaspoon Honey
Any Flavored Oil to Taste
1 Vitamin E Capsule (as a preservative) (optional)

Honey Balm
Ingredients:
3 oz. Almond Oil
2 Teaspoons Honey
1/2 oz. Beeswax or Beeswax Pellets
1 Vitamin E Capsule (as a preservative)
1-4 Drops Essential Oil

Almond Lip Gloss
Ingredients:
2 Teaspoons Grated Beeswax or Beeswax Pellets
3 - 6 Drops Flavored Oil
1 Teaspoon Sweet Almond Oil
3 Drops Honey
1 1/2 Teaspoon Cocoa Butter
1 Vitamin E Capsule (as a preservative)

Helps heal cold sores.
Ingredients:
1 oz. Emu Oil
1 oz. Almond Oil
1 oz. Avocado Oil
1/2 oz. Shaved Beeswax or Beeswax Pellets
1/4 oz. Aloe Vera Gel
6 Drops Lavender Essential Oil
2 Drops Tea Tree Essential Oil
3 Drops Lime Essential Oil

Honey Lip Balm
Ingredients:
2 tsp. olive oil
1/2 tsp. beeswax
1/2 tsp. cocoa butter
1/2 tsp. honey
3 drops essential oil (I like orange.)
1 vitamin E capsule
Measure oil, beeswax and cocoa butter into a glass or enamel pan. Melt over low heat. A hotplate works well and reduces the risk of overheating the oils. Stir the mixture often until the wax is melted. Remove from heat and stir in the honey and essential oil. Pinch opens the vitamin E capsule and squeezes the contents into the mixture. Stir well. Pour the mixture into containers.

Aloe Vera Lip Gloss
Ingredients:
1 tsp Aloe Vera gel
1/2 tsp coconut oil
1 tsp petroleum jelly
Mix the ingredients in a glass bowl, and microwave for 1 - 2 minutes.
Pour into container.

Vaseline Lip Balm
Ingredients:
3 parts Vaseline
1 part beeswax

Flavoring
Mix well

Chocolate Balm

3 Tbsp. Cocoa Butter
4-5 Chocolate Chips
1 capsule, Vitamin E
Melt and blend ingredients with a spoon until smooth, put into a container and refrigerate until solid.

Vanilla Lip Gloss

Ingredients:
1 tablespoon grates beeswax
1/2 tablespoon coconut oil
1/8 teaspoon vitamin E oil
1/8 teaspoon vanilla extract
Slowly melt beeswax, coconut oil, and vitamin E oil
Stir in the vanilla extract then cool

Vanilla Lip Balm

Ingredients:
1 TBL Petroleum Jelly
1 TBL Aloe Vera Gel
1 1/2 tsp coconut oil
1/2 tsp vanilla
Heat in double boiler (or microwave) then pour into container to cool.

Candle Wax Lip Balm

Ingredients:
½ teaspoon candle wax (melted)
2 teaspoons of Olive Oil
½ teaspoon of Shea Butter or you can also add Cocoa Butter
½ teaspoon of Honey and any flavor of oil to taste
One vitamin E capsule to preserve the Lip Balm

Eye shadow Lip Balm

Take an eye shadow break it up and mix it with Vaseline or beeswax.

For a glossy shine, use an iridescent or glittery eye shadow. White/silver/grey glossies are best.

Cocoa Butter Lip Gloss
Ingredients:
1/2 tsp grated Beeswax
1 tsp cocoa butter
1 tsp almond oil or olive
Melt all together by means of water bath (put in a cup & set in sink of hot water) and then put into a lip balm container

Castor Oil Lip Balm
Ingredients:
3 oz castor oil
1.5 oz cocoa butter
1.5 oz beeswax
Melt in microwave. Add oil. Stir. Pour into containers.

Sweet Balm/Gloss
Ingredients:
2 tsp beeswax
1 tsp honey
7 tsp castor oil or jojoba or sweet almond oil
1/8 tsp. Flavor oil
Melt the oil and beeswax together in a little pan over low heat until the beeswax is melted. Take off the stove and then add in your honey and whisk it all together. When the mixture is nearly cool add in your flavor oil, mix it up again and then pour into your lip balm container. Since this comes out to be more like a gloss you can always add more beeswax to it so that it is a little harder. Maybe another 1/2 tsp would do it.

Heal Sores Balm
Ingredients:
3 oz almond oil
2 tsp pure honey
1/2 oz beeswax
1 tsp tea tree oil
Melt all together and stir while cooling.

Quick & Easy Lip Balm
Spoon full of Vaseline in a cup (you don't even need to heat it).
Add some honey (depending on how sweet you want it).
Mix together or whip. Lip sticks color shavings for color.
To solidify faster after putting it in a container, submerse it in a cup
of ice water or put it in the freezer until solid.

Hemp Oil Lip Balm
Ingredients:
3 Tbsp coconut oil
1 Tbsp castor oil
1 Tbsp sunflower oil
1 Tbsp hemp seed oil
1 Tbsp beeswax
1 Tbsp honey
Essential Oil to taste (I use peppermint)
Melt the wax, and coconut oil together (I use the microwave) Add
the honey and heat a little. Stir constantly and add your sunflower
and castor oil. As the mixture begins to thicken add the hempseed
oil and your choice of essential oil. STIR CONTANTLY until it
thickens.

Peppermint Lip Balm
Ingredients:
2 Tbsp petroleum jelly
1 tsp beeswax
10-14 drops peppermint essential oil
In a small pot, melt the petroleum jelly, and then add beeswax.
When melted, remove from heat and add peppermint essential oil.
Pour into a lip pot and cool.

Nude Lip Balm Trendy
Ingredients:
1/4 tsp. of Aloe Vera lotion
1/4 tsp. of your color of foundation
1 tbsp. of Vaseline
Mix together in a small bowl with a cotton swab.
You can even skip the Aloe Vera lotion if you want.

Fruity Lip Gloss --Made with Kool-Aid!
Ingredients:
2 tbsp. solid shortening
1 tbsp. fruit-flavored powdered drink mix (Kool-Aid)
35 mm plastic film container
Mix shortening and drink mix together in a small microwave-safe container until smooth. Place container in the microwave on high for 30 seconds until mixture becomes a liquid. Pour the mixture into a plastic film container or any other type of small airtight container. Place the fruity lip gloss mixture in the refrigerator for 20 to 30 minutes or until firm.

Cinnamon Lip Gloss
2 tablespoons petroleum jelly
1/4 teaspoon lipstick, any color
4 drops cinnamon oil
Place petroleum jelly in small microwave container. Top with lipstick. Microwave for
20-30 seconds on High power (100%) or until mixture has softened. Blend well. Mix in cinnamon.

Hard Candy Lip Gloss
Ingredients:
2 Tbsp petroleum jelly
1 tsp beeswax
2-3 pieces of your favorite hard candy (jolly ranchers work great!)
In a small pot (or microwave), melt the petroleum jelly, hard candy and beeswax.
Pour into a lip container and cool.
In a microwave, melt about eight chocolate chips with about four tablespoons of cocoa butter and 1/4 teaspoon of olive oil. Stir at 20-second intervals until the chocolate melts and the product are well mixed. Place in small containers and refrigerate until hardened. Use as needed. Makes a great gift, too!

Cocoa Butter Minty Lip Balm
Ingredients:
1-1/2 parts cocoa butter

1-1/2 parts grated beeswax
3 parts edible vegetable oil of your choice (almond, apricot kernel, avocado, extra virgin olive, hemp seed, jojoba, Coconut, macadamia nut, castor all work well... but keep in mind if you plan on selling lip balm or giving as a gift, that some people are allergic to nut oils). Spearmint and/or peppermint flavoring oil Melt the cocoa butter and beeswax slowly and carefully in a microwave, or over a double boiler on the stove until melted. Add oil and stir well. Add spearmint or peppermint flavoring oils, or both, a few drops at a time, to taste. Gently reheat if needed. Cool slightly before pouring into containers. To test consistency, place a drop on a spoon and set in the refrigerator to cool for a few minutes. Test on your lips. For a softer lip balm, add more oil. For a harder lip balm, add more beeswax.

Chocolate Lip Gloss
Ingredients:
1 1/2 tsp grated cocoa butter
1/2 tsp coconut oil
1/8 tsp vitamin E oil
1/4 tsp grated chocolate or 3 small chocolate chips
In a double boiler or microwave heat the cocoa butter, coconut oil, and vitamin E oil until melted. Stir in the chocolate chips and keep stirring until melted and well blended Pour into small container and allow cooling before using

Beeswax Lip Balm
Ingredients:
2 tablespoons beeswax
1 tablespoon coconut oil
Melt the ingredients over a double boiler. Pour into a container while still hot
Since it will harden as it cools.

Cocoa Butter Minty Lip Balm
Ingredients:
1-1/2 parts cocoa butter
1-1/2 parts grated beeswax

3 parts edible vegetable oil of your choice (almond, apricot kernel, avocado, extra virgin olive, hemp seed, jojoba, coconut, macadamia nut, castor all work well... but keep in mind if you plan on selling lip balm or giving as a gift, that some people are allergic to nut oils) Spearmint and/or peppermint flavoring oil.

Melt the cocoa butter and beeswax slowly and carefully in a microwave, or over a double boiler on the stove until melted. Add oil and stir well. Add spearmint or peppermint flavoring oils, or both, a few drops at a time, to taste. Gently reheat if needed. Cool slightly before pouring into containers. To test consistency, place a drop on a spoon and set in the refrigerator to cool for a few minutes. Test on your lips. For a softer lip balm, add more oil. For a harder lip balm, add more beeswax.

Cassandra Green
Sugar Leg Wax
Ingredients:
2 cups sugar
1/4 C lemon juice
1/4 C water
2 tbsp vegetable glycerin
Waxing cloth strips (buy at the drugstore) OR use strips of linen cut to the size of these strips wooden Popsicle sticks (to stir the wax and to apply) combine all ingredients in a saucepan. Stir frequently while heating to 250 degrees F or softball stage. Pour into jars and cover with lids. If you use plastic jars, you'll be able to microwave this mixture instead of heating it on the stove. That's it!! You just mad your own leg wax/sugar that you'd pay $20 for in the stores!

To use the Sugar Wax: Heat in the microwave for ten seconds on high. Using a wooden stir stick, stir VERY well. It should be warm but not HOT. Please be very careful when heating up this wax - it's very easy to burn yourself. If the wax isn't warm enough, place it back in the microwave for five seconds, and stir again. Remember, this is hot sugar syrup- if it gets too hot you'll be badly burned. Lightly powder the area to be treated. Spread a thin layer of the wax on in the same direction as the hair grows. Apply the waxing cloth strip over the applied wax, and rub down well to get the wax to stick to the cloth. Pull your skin taut, and in one quick motion pull the fabric off of your skin AGAINST the direction of hair growth. Continue with the other areas of your leg or wherever you're waxing. When you're done waxing a complete area, rub in lotion, Aloe Vera gel (fresh is best) or oil to soothe your legs. You can use the homemade waxing strips again if you soak it in soapy water to dissolve the sugar off the fabric and then toss it in with your wash as normal.

ABOUT THE AUTHOR

Cassandra Green became interested in natural beauty and natural beauty remedies. Through constant research and experimentation, Cassandra has discovered some amazing tips on natural beauty secrets. She currently lives and works in New York. In her spare time Cassandra writes articles about natural beauty secret on her blog. Cassandra has worked hard to make available help for everyone get the vital information needed to maintain natural beauty.